Integrating Family Planning Training into Medical Education

A Case Study of St. Paul's Hospital Millennium Medical College (SPHMMC), Addis Ababa.

Lia T. Gebremedhin, MD, MHA, Balkachew Nigatu, MD, Delayehu Bekele, MD, MPH, Senait Fisseha, MD, JD, Berhanu G. Gebremeskel, MD, MPH

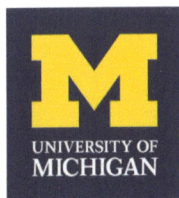

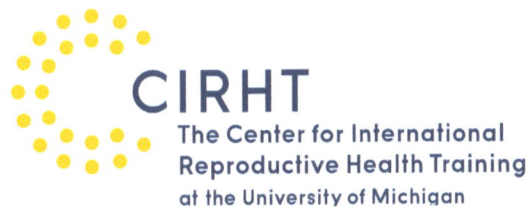

UNIVERSITY OF MICHIGAN

CIRHT
The Center for International
Reproductive Health Training
at the University of Michigan

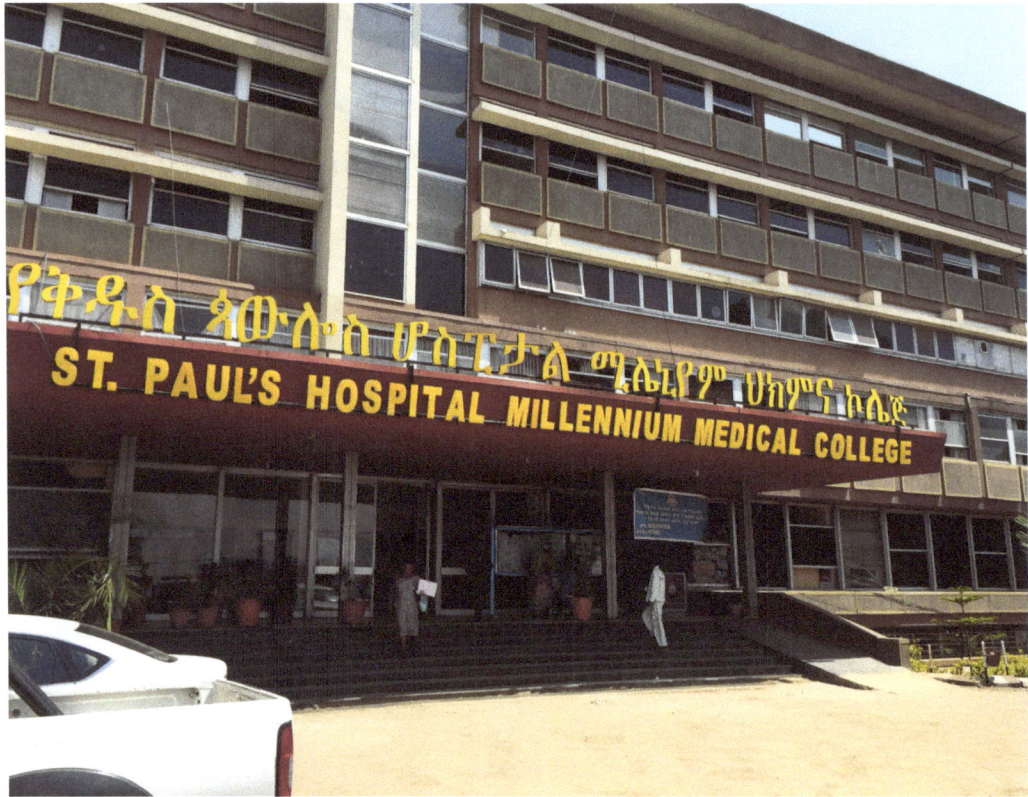

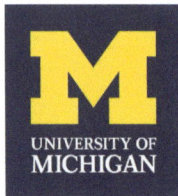

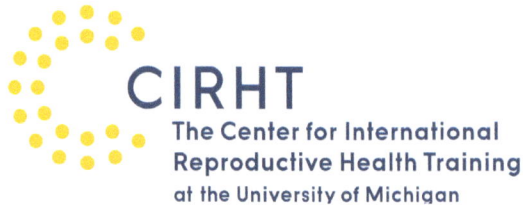

Published in the United States of America by
Michigan Publishing
Manufactured in the United States of America

ISBN 978-1-60785-402-9 (paper)

Contents

Acknowledgments   v

Executive Summary   vii

I. Introduction   1

II. Methodology   3

III. Why St. Paul's and U-of-M?   3

IV. Why Integration in Pre-Service Training?   4

V. What Were the Pillars for the Success of the Program?   5

    1. Competency-Based Curriculum Integration   5

    What Is the Approach?   5

    What Happened after Graduation?   7

    2. Faculty Development Initiatives   10

    3. Service and Systems Improvement   13

    Michu Clinic   13

    Quality Improvement   15

    4. Supportive College Leadership   16

VI. Lessons Learned   17

References   19

Acknowledgments

We would like to express our gratitude to the faculty and leadership of St. Paul's Hospital Millennium Medical College in Addis Ababa and the University of Michigan. Our sincere thanks goes to all the trainees, medical students, interns, and residents who participated in this innovative program and willingly provided their feedback through surveys and interviews, which provided the basis for the content of this report.

We are grateful for the Ministry of Health of the Federal Democratic Republic of Ethiopia for its commitment to family planning and comprehensive abortion care and for creating a conducive environment for the pre-service integration program to be successfully implemented at St. Paul's.

This case study was made possible through the generous financial support of an anonymous donor through the Center for International Reproductive Health Training (CIRHT) at the University of Michigan.

The authors gratefully acknowledge the editorial support of Michigan Publishing.

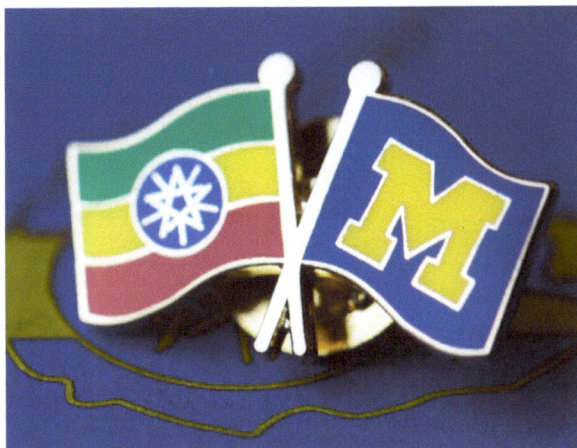

Executive Summary

Ethiopia has made considerable progress in increasing the uptake of family planning and comprehensive abortion services (FP/CAC) in the last decade owing to, among others, the Ministry of Health's commitment in making family planning a national health priority, its favorable national policies and strategies, including the Health Extension Program, and the effort to increase the availability of family planning commodities across all tiers of the health system. However, there is still a substantial level of unmet need for contraception, and unsafe abortions continue to contribute to high maternal mortality in Ethiopia. One of the shortcomings of traditional medical training programs in the country was not incorporating these all-important competencies in providing contraception and safe abortion. This was posited to be one of the factors that resulted in medical graduates who did not have sound attitudes, and a sentiment to instead relegate these services to middle- and low-level health professionals.

The Obstetrics and Gynecology (OBGYN) faculty at St. Paul's Hospital Millennium Medical College (SPHMMC) in Addis Ababa, in partnership with Dr. Senait Fisseha at University of Michigan (U-M), saw this as a missed opportunity and designed and implemented a program in pre-service integration of FP/CAC services beginning with the first class of St. Paul's interns in 2012, following a baseline assessment that confirmed the lack of these competencies in the soon-to-be graduates. This competency-based training is hands-on and simulation-supported, incorporating leadership and advocacy training as well as a dedicated rotation time in a family planning unit during the trainee's internship in OBGYN.

The underlying approach in the partnership was based on sustainability and anchored in faculty capacity building and reproductive health service improvement. The partnership between St. Paul's and U-M concurrently incorporated this integration from the inception phase of the OBGYN residency program.

Following the graduation of St. Paul's first class, the pre-service integration has become a standard part of medical training for St. Paul's trainees. A total of 216 medical students were successfully trained in rigorous, hands-on, competency-based modality in FP/CAC and have expressed their satisfaction with the program and how it has increased their competency and confidence in providing these services and made them become better, more compassionate doctors. Graduates of the program, who are deployed to various corners of the country, have become skilled providers of these services, champions for the cause of women's health, and leaders who mentor and supervise other health care providers in their facility and satellite sites. St. Paul's OBGYN department has drawn a large number of exceptional OBGYN faculty who are training an ever-increasing cohort of bright residents and medical students. Currently there are 16 faculty members, up from 2 at the inception of the partnership in 2011; St. Paul's now has the highest number of OBGYNs in the public sector anywhere in the country, training 63 residents, 65 interns, and 180 clinical-year medical student in integrated, competency-based curricula that substantially emphasize contraception and comprehensive abortion care.

U-M faculty regularly support the development of faculty and residents at SPHMMC in different clinical and teaching skills and research. Their research support encompasses research methodology trainings and one-on-one mentorship, which has resulted in scholarly reproductive health publications and presentations in major international conferences. The quality and volume of contraception and safe abortion services at St. Paul's Hospital have shown a sustained growth over the last four years, further reinforced with the launch of a newly redesigned woman-friendly reproductive health clinic and several on-going quality-improvement initiatives spearheaded by committed faculty, which are paving the way to making St. Paul's a Center of Excellence (CoE) for reproductive health both nationally and in the region.

The SPHMMC–U-M partnership's integration of FP/CAC, faculty development, and service improvement has resulted in an unprecedented advancement in training, service provision, and research capacity over the last several years and is creating confident, competent, compassionate physicians who are providing these services and mentoring fellow health professionals. The demonstrable success of the pre-service integration is now being scaled up to eight other medical schools in the country through the Center for International Reproductive Health Training (CIRHT) at the University of Michigan. This model will be subsequently expanded to other Sub-Saharan African and South East Asian countries with high rates of maternal mortality and unmet need for FP/CAC services.

I. Introduction

Family planning and the provision of safe and comprehensive abortion services are the cornerstone of public health strategy to avert the huge toll of maternal morbidity and mortality associated with unintended pregnancies and unsafe abortions, while access to those services is a key element of the sexual and reproductive health rights of women.[1-5] Several investigators have also documented the impact of this approach on development as highlighted by the *"demographic dividend."*[4] The government of Ethiopia has underscored the strategy of increasing the uptake of family planning services nationally as part and parcel of economic development and the improvement of the health status of the population. The ministry of health has long identified the importance of FP/CAC and made it one of the pillars of the national health focus. Multifaceted approaches to improve access to family planning such as the Health Extension Program, improved availability of contraception and safe abortion services at all levels of the health system, and improved laws and policies have all been key to the achievement garnered so far.[6,7] This is demonstrated in the reduction of deaths from unsafe abortions from 30% to 6%–9% following the implementation of the revised abortion law in 2005, and the improved contraceptive prevalence rate (CPR) of 42% from 15% (among married women) in 2005.[6,8-16] Despite all these efforts and progress so far, Ethiopia still suffers from an unmet need for family planning at 25%, with an estimated 41% of unintended pregnancies, and a high rate of unsafe abortions resulting in a maternal mortality ratio of 420 for every 100,000 live births, making Ethiopia's level among the highest in the world.[9,15]

One of the potential contributors to this gap is that in academic medical centers across the country, adequate attention has not been given to training health professionals who are well versed in providing a full range of comprehensive reproductive health services. Traditionally, these services were relegated to low- and midlevel health care providers who generally acquired these skills through in-service training, while physicians had only a minimal role. The major reason posited for this sentiment has been the lack of adequate hands-on training in family planning methods and the provision of comprehensive abortion care for medical doctors during their training in medical school. In the last decade, Ethiopia has undergone an accelerated expansion in the number of medical schools, a leap from 3 to 27 public medical schools. After one year of rotating internships during the last year of medical school, general practitioners who graduate from medical schools in Ethiopia are generally deployed all over the country to render medical services as well as enter into leadership roles in health facilities for at least two to four years before they join residency training. Despite this rapid increase in the workforce, the curriculum in these medical schools was not providing the students adequate skills to be competent providers in comprehensive reproductive health (RH) care apart from one to three hours of didactic lectures on family planning and abortion. Wherever the graduates were posted in the various corners of the country, they were not prepared to provide these RH services and were unable to supervise and lead the team of nurses and other midlevel medical professionals who were providing these RH services. This was noted as a huge missed opportunity by the OBGYN faculty at SPHMMC and Dr. Senait Fisseha, a professor of OBGYN and a reproductive endocrinologist from the University of Michigan (U-M) Dr. Senait is Ethiopian in origin and has a strong passion for women's health. With a commitment to give back to her country, she started spearheading the collaboration between St. Paul's Hospital Millennium Medical College in Addis Ababa and the University of Michigan in 2011.[17] Having underscored the importance of integrating family planning and comprehensive abortion care (FP/CAC) training into the pre-service education as a feasible, sustainable, and cost-effective approach, St. Paul's Hospital Millennium Medical College started piloting this program starting with the first cohort of SPHMMC medical students in 2012 in partnership with the U-M through the support of an anonymous donor.[18,19] The program was successfully implemented in the first group and has now become the standard curriculum; subsequent graduates have acquired competencies in FP/CAC that have translated into the provision of comprehensive care for women in all the places the graduates have been deployed to. The same integration was also applied to the OBGYN residency training program, from inception in 2012 with the collaboration of the U-M.

> "You cannot implement U.S. standards in Ethiopia, but a U.S. institution with experience in Africa really has more to deliver in Africa."
>
> **DR. TEDROS ADHANOM GEBREYESUS**

This case study sets out to examine and document the successful implementation and the broader impact of this unique and innovative program of integrated pre-service training in family planning and comprehensive abortion care in medical education and OBGYN resident education at SPHMMC in Addis Ababa, in partnership with the U-M. The findings and lessons learned from the program have enabled the replication and scale-up of pre-service training in other Ethiopian medical schools through CIRHT, and we believe the detailed accounts of this case study might help expand efforts beyond Ethiopia.

II. Methodology

A mixed methods approach was used to chronicle the success story, mainly through structured key-informant interviews and desk reviews. Additionally, we collected relevant information garnered from prior workshops, progress reports, and presentations at international conferences. Historical data about St. Paul's Hospital are gathered from the hospital leadership and publicly available domains.

III. Why St. Paul's and U-of-M?

SPHMMC was established as a medical school in 2007 by the Ethiopian federal Ministry of Health under the initiative of Dr. Tedros Adhanom Gebreyesus (the then minister of health) with the objective of producing health professionals who are both competent and committed to serving their nation using a unique modular and integrated curriculum.

"It started as a school with a different path; a pathfinder in its own right" says Dr. Tedros, who is currently the minister of foreign affairs in Ethiopia.[17] SPHMMC recruits students who have completed high school, but unlike any other medical school in Ethiopia, it selects its own students through interviews and exams to ensure the candidates not only are academically bright but also have the motivation to serve. Dr. Zerihun Abebe, provost of SPHMMC, captures St. Paul's ambitious visions as follows: *"It's a small medical school with a very big potential."*

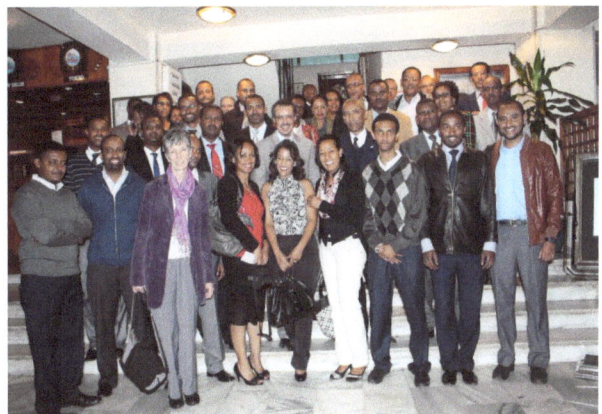

Launching of OBGYN residency with Dr. Tedros Adhanom, Dr. Senait Fisseha, leadership and faculty of St. Paul's, first cohort of residents, and other invited guests

By the end of 2011, at the invitation of Dr. Senait Fisseha, Dr. Tedros Adhanom had the opportunity to visit the U-M, and after seeing the successful and long-standing global health partnership they have built with Ghana through the leadership of Dr. Timothy Johnson, chair of the OBGYN department, he asked U-M to start a similar partnership at SPHMMC especially geared toward improving maternal health given the stark need. *"You cannot implement U.S. standards in Ethiopia, but a U.S. institution with experience in Africa really has more to deliver in Africa. They have the experience, so they will come with the right understanding and come with something that is tailor made for you."* Dr. Tedros said.[20] Soon after Dr. Tedros's visit, a team from U-M that included Dr. Timothy Johnson, Dr. Senait Fisseha, and a representative from the Center of Global Health at the U-M, as well as Dr. Richard Adanu from the University of Ghana, went to visit SPHMMC and connected with Dr. Lia Tadesse, who was the vice provost of SPHMMC at the time. Within a short time, the collaboration kicked off by launching a residency training program in OBGYN at SPHMMC in 2012, which became an excellent platform for the integration of family planning into pre-service training.

IV. Why Integration in Pre-Service Training?

Faced with the gap in competency based training in family planning and comprehensive abortion care in the medical school curriculums, faculty members in the department of OBGYN at St. Paul's and Dr. Senait Fisseha embarked on workable approaches to address this missed opportunity for the newly founded medical college under the very supportive leadership of Provost Dr. Mesfin Araya and Vice Provost Dr. Lia Tadesse. This gap in training was confirmed by a baseline assessment conducted by the SPHMMC OBGYN faculty to determine the knowledge and skill base of the first batch of 38 interns in September 2012.[18,21] One of the startling findings of this basic evaluation was that none of the interns at that time had ever performed the insertion or removal of a birth control implant or an intrauterine device (IUD), with less than a quarter of the inaugural class having observed an implant insertion.

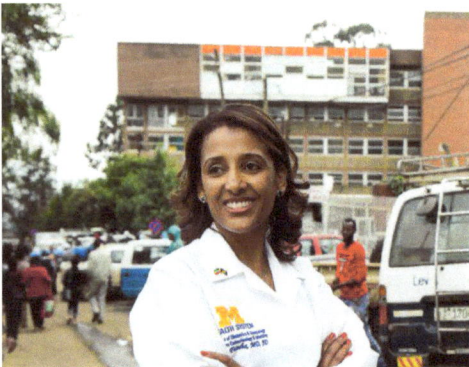

The approach of integrating family planning and comprehensive abortion care training into pre-service training of undergraduate medical students was borne out of the several benefits that it has over the traditional in-service education that has been used in the country for several decades.

The following potential benefits of pre-service education over in-service training were considered:

"I would like St. Paul's to be the premier institution in Ethiopia, if not in East Africa."

DR. SENAIT FISSEHA

- Pre-service training is a cost-effective and efficient strategy, reaching a large number of trainees at a time.
- It provides the time necessary to produce competent physicians capable of delivering patient-centered care with a sound attitude.
- It mainstreams FP/CAC service delivery and avoids compartmentalization.
- It allows the faculty to model behavior for the trainees.
- It facilitates fitting new graduates into the health system, which improves performance.

V. What Were the Pillars for the Success of the Program?

1. Competency-Based Curriculum Integration

The program of integration in pre-service training is modeled after the competency-based curriculum of the Ryan Residency Training Program in Abortion and Family Planning in the United States, with adjustments made to fit the Ethiopian context.

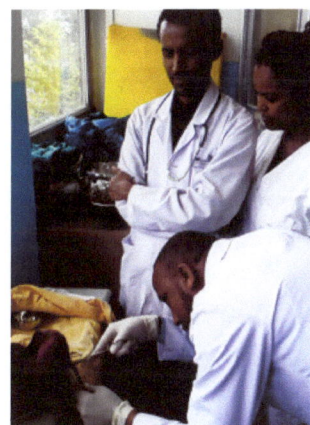

SPHMMC students practicing on a PPIUD (postpartum IUD) model

There is an emphasis on practical skills above and beyond theory-driven approaches that used to be conducted through didactic lectures. Traditionally, there was a dearth of hands-on experience, and the time allotted for family planning rarely exceeded one to two lecture hours throughout a student's time in the medical school. Due to the lack of a rigorous training in skills acquisition, the previous graduates from medical schools in Ethiopia were less interested in and less confident about delivering the much-needed RH services. It was evident that these physicians were not very involved in family planning service provision in the communities that they were assigned to.

What Is the Approach?

With particular focus on competency-based training, the curriculum incorporates a blend of the following methods to ensure that trainees will have all the necessary skills to deliver a full suite of RH services:

- Didactic lectures, seminars, and tutorials that give students the evidence and theoretical base for FP/CAC and include relevant epidemiology during Clinical I and II years (CI and CII)
- Case-based scenarios that illustrate a particular facet of FP and/or CAC
- Simulation-based training on models that encourages the acquisition of skills such as long-acting reversible contraception (LARC) methods (e.g., IUD, birth control implant) and surgical abortion (e.g., Manual Vacuum Aspiration [MVA]) in their CII year
- Dedicated time (one week) for interns to spend in the family planning unit during their OBGYN attachment, providing FP/CAC services for clients under supervision
- Periodic objective assessment of acquired skills by tallying procedures observed and/or performed into a log book that is duly signed by a supervising resident or faculty member

"Previously there may have been a one-hour lecture, and then [we] memorize the information that we blurt out in an exam, and then we forget it. With this program, we have additional training and hands-on practice."

DR. AHMED IBRAHIM, GRADUATE OF SPHMMC

- Training on the legal aspects of abortion and counseling using the national training manual
- Training in leadership, advocacy, and values clarification to improve attitude and professionalism (particular focus is given to this training)
- Students assessments where FP/CAC is given due emphasis and included in the theoretical and practical examination/assessments, with at least two stations dedicated for FP/CAC in CI and CII OSCE (Objective Structured Clinical Exam)

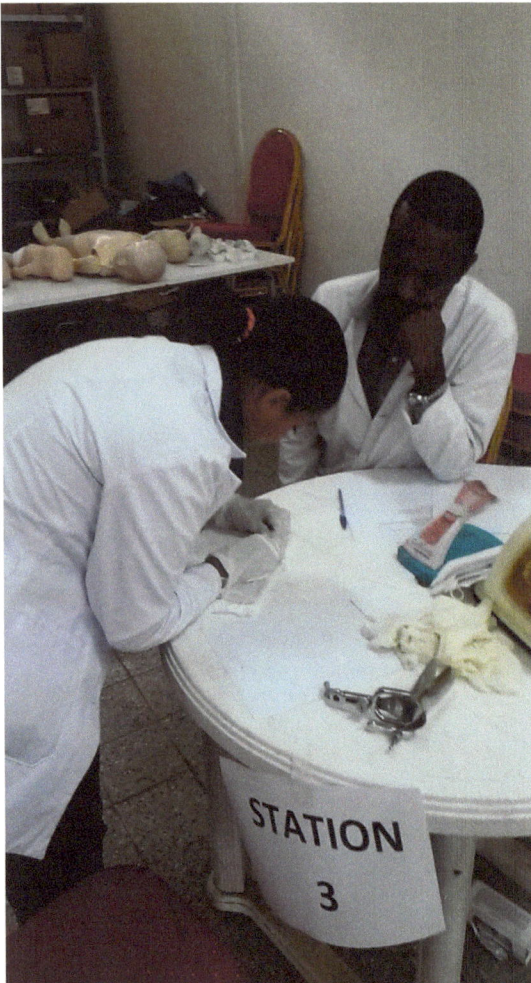

SPHMMC student being assessed on IUD insertion at an OSCE station

The OBGYN residency curriculum at SPHMMC was designed to incorporate family planning and abortion training from the development phase of the program, with a one-month family planning rotation required each year over the first three years of residency. Incorporating family planning–based training has made the residents remarkably competent in providing comprehensive RH services and carrying out their clinical services with admirable professionalism. Because of this approach, it was possible to ensure the presence of at least one resident in the family planning unit every month and thus had the added benefit of assuring quality care for clients and patients who come to the unit seeking services. Additionally, the residents serve as mentors for the interns and medical students that rotate through the family planning unit. *"Service and training integration in family planning and comprehensive abortion care has changed the mindsets of faculty. As students expand their skills, the faculty have been able to learn more and realize the importance of their leadership in providing comprehensive care to women,"* says Dr. Malede Birara, former chair of OBGYN at SPHMMC.

When SPHMMC was about to launch the implementation of this integrated curriculum, the first batch of students had already started their internship years. Given that the opportune time for this would be with soon-to-be graduates, a package with a modified approach comprising the following was given as an intervention in collaboration with Ipas Ethiopia:

- Two-day, intensive hands-on training on LARC and abortion care at the beginning of their rotation in OBGYN, and
- One-week placement in the family planning unit

Assessment of the outcome of such a training package was done through a review of the log books that tallied the number of procedures the trainees performed before their graduation and the results of a self-administered survey. The overwhelming majority (96%) of the graduates indicated that the training they received was excellent/good, all the graduating class had inserted implants, and 93% had removed them. Potentially owing to the low uptake of IUDs by women, two-thirds inserted IUDs during their internship years and a quarter performed IUD removals.[18,21]

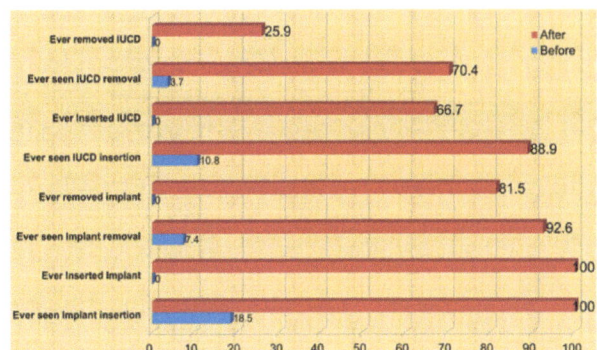

Results of the assessment of procedures observed and/or performed before and after the first FP/CAC training

Subsequent to the graduation of the first class, more medical students have passed through the training, with the training being integrated starting in their CI attachments with both didactic and hands-on training mentioned above, which continues to increase the skill base of the students. Students speak passionately about the invaluable experience and confidence they are gaining with the integrated curriculum, which emphasizes hands-on training and simulations. The students and residents also agree that the counseling skills built through this program are crucial and that these skills are making them better doctors.

The training is not limited to skill and knowledge acquisition but also incorporates a leadership and advocacy training that has been delivered by a local institution, the Center for African Leadership Studies (CALS), in addition to the values clarification session they receive through the program. Overall, the training has demonstrated a visible difference in the caliber of medical graduates of SPHMMC, with most of them taking on a variety of leadership roles and spearheading reform initiatives in the institutions they are assigned to all over the country. *"If I get a phone call from a graduate of SPHMMC, 90% of the time it is about improving the health system,"* says Dr. Keseteberhan Admasu, current minister of health of Ethiopia.

What Happened after Graduation?

Postdeployment refresher training on FP/CAC and leadership was given in Addis Ababa a year after the first group of graduates had been practicing in their respective health facilities. This was an excellent platform for graduates to learn from each other by sharing their experiences on both the successes and the challenges they were facing, and it was used as an opportunity to interview 35 of the first 38 graduates of SPHMMC. Of that first class, 60% (21/35) were providing both safe abortion and contraception services, with a total of 71.4% (25/35) of graduates providing long-acting reversible contraception (LARC) and/or safe abortion services, while 11.4% (4/35) were delivering long-term contraception without safe abortion services due to moral and/or religious dilemma. Of the 28.6% (10/35) that were not providing any of these services, the majority attributed lack of necessary supplies and equipment as the number one barrier to service provision, showing there is still work to be done to improve access to family planning nationwide. Other barriers to providing abortion services cited included unsupportive environment, fear of stigma, and a need to refresh skills. The second batch of St. Paul's graduates has subsequently participated in family planning refresher workshop and leadership training before deployment to their respective health facilities.

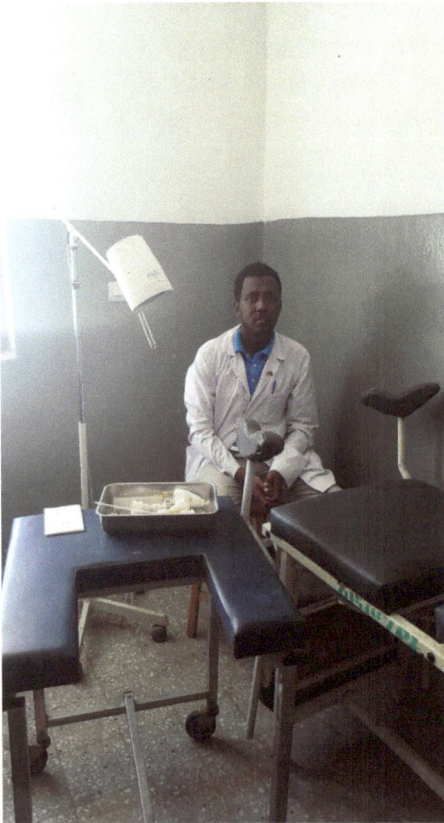

Dr. Kasim in the renovated abortion clinic at Assaita Hospital FP/CAC training

Dr. Kasim Ibrahim, a 26-year-old general practitioner who was among the first graduates of SPHMMC in 2013, was assigned as a medical director soon after he started working at Assaita Hospital in the Afar region. Upon assuming his leadership position, Dr. Kasim made it his life's mission to improve the health care delivered to the population the hospital serves, with particular focus on maternal and child health.

The Afar region is one of the four underdeveloped, emerging regions in Ethiopia where most of the health indicators are very poor, marked by a huge lack of human resources for health and infrastructure. By marshaling resources from within the region and from the federal Ministry of Health and other donor agencies, the young and energetic Dr. Kasim indicates that maternal health is *"a critical focus point"* for him. Some of the changes he has brought about include introducing family planning and abortion care services to the hospital and improving the knowledge and attitude in the community served. Midwives in his facility are also trained to counsel all postpartum women on family planning. On average, around 10–20 contraceptive implants are inserted every month in an area where these issues are very sensitive. Both medical abortion and MVA are being provided currently, which were not available before he took over.

The abortion care room at Assaita Hospital has been completely renovated and fitted with the necessary equipment to support the optimal delivery of services. Additionally, Dr. Kasim oversees the training of health care providers in FP/CAC in the three adjoining health centers.

Dr. Kasim proudly states, *"The family planning and leadership trainings I had in my days at SPHMMC have enabled me to lead the reform in the remotely located and underresourced district hospital in an organized manner."* He has a deep commitment to care for every woman and child and says, *"I won't stop providing care as long as I am alive!"*

"My passion to give women-centered care comes from the training I received as a medical student at SPHMMC, which has made me a confident professional and [one who can] even pass my knowledge and skills to providers in hospitals I am assigned in as well as to satellite health centers." says Dr. Ayantu Tesfaye, also of the first batch of SPHMMC graduates. Dr. Ayantu is posted in Ambo Hospital in the Oromia region, the largest and most

populous region in the nation, where she is providing a variety of reproductive health care services, including FP/CAC services, as a result of the program in integrated FP/CAC training at SPHMMC. Since her placement as a general practitioner, the hospital has seen a substantial growth in the use of long-acting reversible contraceptive (LARC) methods. A mean of 15%–17% of women who delivered at the hospital received IUDs, and 191 IUDs or implants were inserted over a period of six months, from July to December of 2014, which was a huge leap from the previous years' data. *"By providing family planning for a woman and preventing unintended pregnancies, my goal is to help [create] happy families. I am proud of serving my own people by choice."*

Dr. Ayantu also provides mentorship and supervision in FP/CAC and HIV treatment for the surrounding health centers. She led an outreach program in March 2015 in Shenen, one of the satellite health centers, during which 170 IUDs were inserted. In the other four health centers, after training the health professionals and carrying out health education for patients, the use of long-acting family planning methods compared to short-term family planning methods had increased substantially. *"The changes I observe in these satellite facilities are my motivations to keep working there."* She presented her work as a physician and mentor for the satellite centers in increasing the uptake of LARC, on a preformed panel at the 2016 International Conference on Family Planning (ICFP) in Indonesia, which was lauded highly by the audience.

"Integration of family planning and abortion training into pre-service education is a feasible approach that sustainably improves the competency of medical students to provide those services," said Dr. Delayehu Bekele, one of SPHMMC's OBGYN faculty when he presented about the program at the 2016 ICFP in Indonesia.

The value of the partnership was not one sided. Supported by different programs at the U-M, medical students and residents as well as public health students from the U-M have been traveling to St. Paul's to engage in different clinical and research activities, pair up with their counterpart students, and be mentored by faculty from SPHMMC and U-M. This helped them gain global health experience, honed their clinical and research skills, enhanced cultural competencies, and broadened their horizons through learning about the different health systems within developing countries like Ethiopia and exploring potential areas of meaningful engagement for their future careers.

> "Saving a mother is everything to her child, so saving a mother is like saving the world of the newborn. If the mother dies, the future of her child dies with it."
>
> **DR. KASIM IBRAHIM, GRADUATE OF SPHMMC**

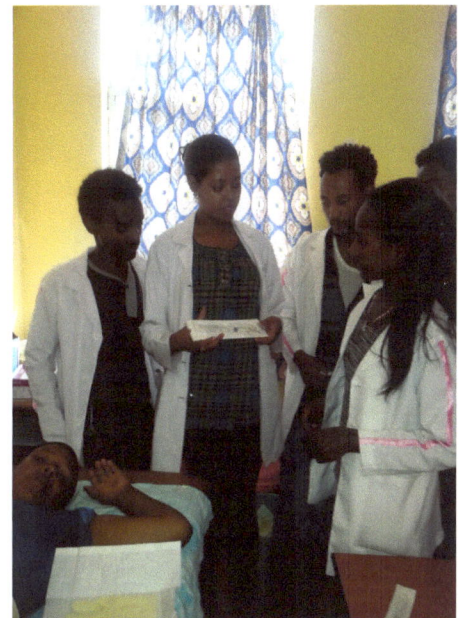

Dr. Ayantu teaching students at Ambo Hospital about IUDs

2. Faculty Development Initiatives

The SPHMMC OBGYN department had only two faculty members when the SPHMMC–U-M collaboration started (the department chair, Dr. Abdulfetah Abdulkadir, and Dr. Lia Tadesse who was working mainly as vice provost) and five when the OBGYN residency was launched in 2012. The strong partnership between U-M and SPHMMC, especially in the areas of faculty development and the potential for growth, has played an instrumental role in drawing many more faculty to SPHMMC. The presence of such committed faculty with the support of their U-M colleagues has been crucial to the successful implementation of the curriculum integration. The OBGYN department has markedly increased its capacity for the 2015–16 academic year, with 16 full-time faculty members training 63 residents, 70 interns, and 180 medical students in their clinical years, with a steep increase in the intake capacity from 7 residents in the first year (2012) to 31 residents admitted in September 2015. The 7 residents who began their training in 2012 graduated in July 2016 and became full-fledged OBGYNs, and they will continue as faculty at SPHMMC, further increasing their numbers. SPHMMC now has the highest number of OBGYNs of any public hospital in Ethiopia.

Cohort/Year	Graduating Interns	Current Residents
1st	38	30
2nd	25	14
3rd	74	12
4th	65	7
Total	**202**	**63**

Total Number of Residents And Interns

SPHMMC OBGYN in 2016 by the Numbers

16 Faculty
63 Residents
70 Interns
180 Clinical Students

Since this program started, University of Michigan faculty have been traveling to Addis Ababa to train and support the teaching faculty at St. Paul's to enhance their skills in delivering competency-based education in reproductive health. U-M OBGYN faculty including Dr. Senait Fisseha, Dr. Carrie Bell, Dr. Jason Bell, Dr. Diana Curran, Dr Beth Skinner, Dr. Suzie As-Sanie, Dr. Carolyn Johnston, Dr. John Randolph, Dr. Tariq Shah and many others have been able to transfer knowledge and skills to their counterparts at St. Paul's and to their residents through hands-on advanced skills training in different areas, including ultrasounds, simulations in immediate postpartum IUDs (PPIUDs), surgical abortion, and laparoscopic tubal ligation. Experienced faculty, such as Dr. Patricia Mullan, have also traveled to SPHMMC to give workshops on medical education and pedagogy and thus enhancing the teaching skills of the faculty.

At the same time, St. Paul's faculty have made several planned trips to the University of Michigan under observer status to learn, among other things, different clinical skills; the structure of educational programs for medical students, residents, and fellows; and the flow of patient-centered care services, research programs, and administration. Two senior residents from SPHMMC also had the

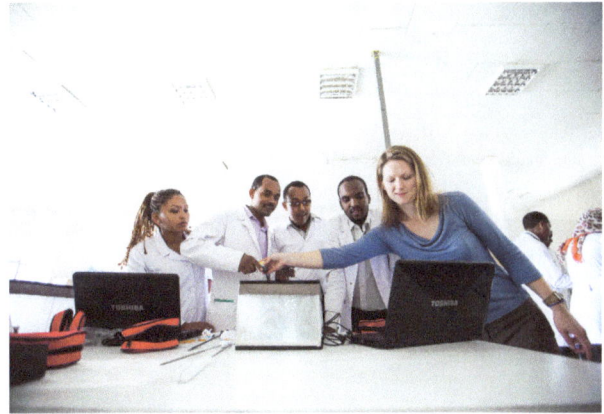

Laparoscopy skills training by U-M faculty member Dr. Skinner at SPHMMC, Addis Ababa

opportunity to gain exposure to OBGYN practices and education in a developed-world setting during a four-week visit to the U-M. This visit broadened their perspectives on high-end obstetrics and gynecology care and supplemented their in-country training.

This has fostered a long-standing partnership between the two institutions, and there is now a very strong ongoing faculty exchange program between U-M and SPHMMC that continues to grow.

The leadership training given through this program was not limited to students; faculty also had the opportunity to participate in the training. With additional funding from American International Health Alliance's (AIHA) Twinning Center, Dr. Balkachew Nigatu, SPHMMC's OBGYN residency program director, received three sequential training courses for program directors through the American College of Obstetricians and Gynecologists (ACOG) in the United States and received certification as a residency director from the CREOG-ACOG (the Council on Resident Education in Obstetrics and Gynecology of the ACOG). This certification training is in addition to the consistent mentoring he receives from Dr. Diana Curran, the U-M OBGYN residency director. His training has not only improved SPHMMC's OBGYN residency program, but as a master trainer, he is

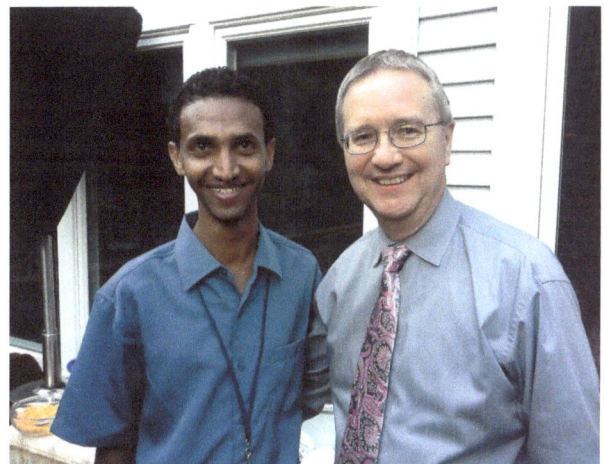

Dr. Ferid Abas, fourth-year SPHMMC resident, visiting U-M with Professor John Randolph

impacting the other residency programs at SPHMMC and will be leading a cascade of trainings for all OBGYN Residency Directors in the various medical schools in Ethiopia. His leadership in the program has helped cultivate a culture of learning, mentoring, and role modeling within the faculty. Dr. Thomas Mekuria, one of the first residents at SPHMMC, says, *"You can talk to your [faculty] mentor at any time. You can go into the surgical theater and do procedures with them and also consult with them on any cases. That's different from the traditional way of teaching in our country because it used to be very distant."*

Systematic and sustainable capacity building in research has also been one of the stalwarts of this program, whereby the research capacity of the faculty and residents has been enriched through periodic training by regularly visiting U-M faculty, who give workshops on research methodology and provide one-on-one mentoring. Dr. Vanessa Dalton, an OBGYN faculty member, together with Sarah Rominiski, a senior research associate, have been supporting and mentoring the residents in their research projects. The research support runs the whole gamut, from helping residents come up with research questions and carrying them through drafting a research protocol, to guiding them toward conducting the particular research projects and focusing on the identified core thematic areas. Of note, three out of the seven in the first batch of residents have selected FP/CAC research projects, and one of the residents has presented his work as a poster at the 2016 ICFP in Indonesia. Professor Richard Adanu, dean of the University of Ghana School of Public Health and editor of the *International Journal of Obstetrics and Gynecology* (IJOG), has also been conducting hands-on research workshops and mentorships, thus forging South–South collaboration for research capacity building. The impact has been demonstrated by the phenomenal research output, with five original articles authored or coauthored by SPHMMC OBGYN faculty published in peer-reviewed medical journals. All seven final-year residents have completed their studies and presented their work. *"The research work of the graduating residents which I reviewed was very impressive, and a few of them can easily get their work published in an international journal,"* says Prof. Richard Adanu.

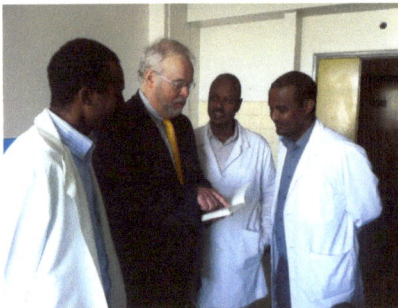

Dr. Timothy Johnson, OBGYN professor and chair of U-M department of OBGYN, with SPHMMC OBGYN faculty (Drs. Balkachew, Mustefa, and Malede), Addis Ababa

Faculty and residents at SPHMMC have had numerous opportunities to network with the OBGYN and family planning community nationally and globally. Several have presented their work in international conferences, which include the International Federation of Gynecology and Obstetrics (FIGO) and International Conference on Family Planning (ICFP).

Along with strengthening the residency and medical student training, the OBGYN department has recently launched a Reproductive Health Fellowship program. This is a two-year subspecialty fellowship program on advanced training in clinical practice, education, and research in family planning, abortion, and other aspects of reproductive health that aims to produce leaders and advocates in family planning and abortion. In addition, through the collaboration with U-M, the department has also commenced fellowships in maternal-fetal medicine, gynecologic oncology, and infertility.

The department, in collaboration with U-M faculty and the Ethiopian Society of OBGYNs (ESOG), is charged with organizing a Continuing Medical Education (CME) lecture series in family planning, safe abortion, and maternal health. These CME series are running almost every year and are well attended by OBGYNs and other RH providers from all over the country.

Building capabilities through developing open educational resources (OER) was another area supported by faculty and staff from the department of the learning health sciences (formerly the department of medical education) and information and communications technology [ICT] at the U-M. SPHMMC faculty and residents have created new, freely available OER designed specifically for their learners and have adapted some resources from previous OER developed by Ghanaian colleagues as well. Some of the materials produced include demonstrations on long-acting contraceptives like implants and IUDs. Setting up a learning resource room with computers, books, and online journals for OBGYN residents and medical students, and developing a robust network infrastructure with capabilities for video conferencing to facilitate remote teaching, was also supported by the program. *"The technology collaboration which started with the creation and delivery of OER for OBGYN has grown to ensure that there is proper ICT infrastructure and digital tools for better training and patient care,"* says Kathleen Omollo, who was leading this support from the U-M.

> "The integrated curriculum at SPHMMC was not started with [an] external push. We were fortunate enough to have dedicated [though few at the beginning], passionate faculty who modeled appropriate behavior. This has helped in starting it right and ensuring continuity. Mind you, every faculty member was on board from the outset—that is the pillar for the success at SPHMMC, with the tremendous guidance of U-M faculty."
>
> **DR. BALKACHEW NIGATU, OBGYN FACULTY AND RESIDENCY DIRECTOR AT SPHMMC**

3. Service and Systems Improvement

Michu Clinic

In general, family planning and safe abortion services were traditionally considered primary care and so very little attention was given to those services in tertiary centers like SPHMMC. When this program started, the family planning unit was a very small room at the back of the outpatient clinic that was not properly catering to the needs of women.

With the goal of improving the quality and accessibility of family planning and abortion services at SPHMMC as part of the integrated

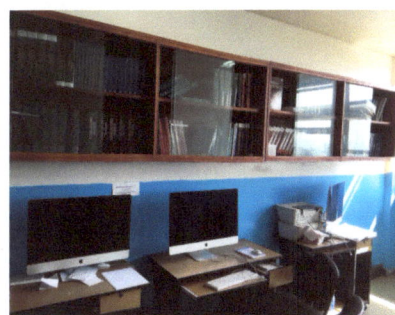

OBGYN Learning Resource Room at SPHMMC

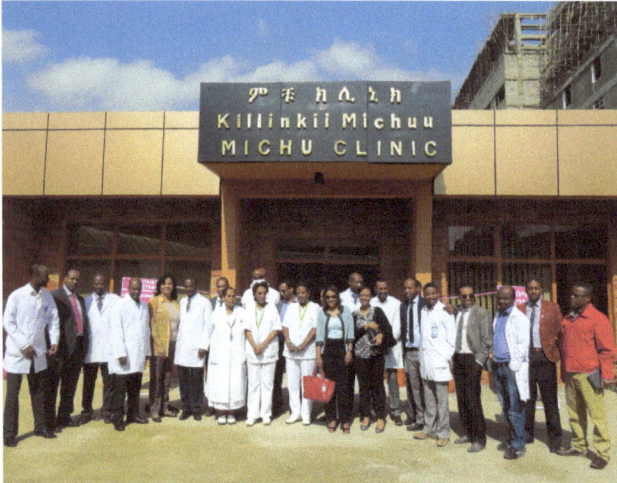

Inauguration of the Michu Clinic at SPHMMC

training program and with the greater vision of making it a National Center of Excellence (CoE) in family planning and abortion training and service, the college leadership and the OBGYN department championed the development of a new RH center.

Thus a newly redesigned, woman-friendly reproductive health unit has been inaugurated at SPHMMC in early January 2016. This spacious center is named Michu Clinic; "Michu" is an Amharic word for "comfortable," that also pays tribute to the partnership with the University of Michigan. The new clinic supports SPHMMC's efforts to meet the nation's growing family planning demands and reflects a commitment to improved access to quality care that puts patients first. With a visible and convenient location at the front of the SPHMMC campus, this center is providing a full-range of services in one place, including counseling, family planning procedures, and safe abortion. Senior OBGYN faculty are assigned in the clinic through rotations to lead, supervise, and teach the team of residents, interns, and nurses assigned there. This center is expected to increase the uptake of these services and pave the way to the realization of SPHMMC's goal of becoming a Center of Excellence in reproductive health in Ethiopia and the region.

Through the program in partnership with U-M, SPHMMC has gone from being an institution that gave very limited services in family planning and safe abortion to provid-

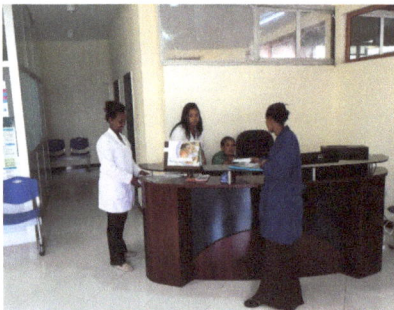

The reception lobby of Michu Clinic at SPHMMC

ing comprehensive services including long-acting reversible contraception (LARC), interval IUDs and postpartum IUDs, birth control implants, and permanent sterilization to comprehensive abortion care, including second-trimester pregnancy termination services. The uptake of family planning and abortion services since the inception of the program has shown a marked rise.

Before the start of the program in 2012, second-trimester abortion services were not available at all, but after the program's inception four years ago, 262 safe second-trimester terminations were provided over a one-year period (July 2014–July 2015), averaging 22 a month. IUD insertions more than tripled, with total contraceptive users rising to 2995 over the same one-year time frame and then to 5071 over the 18-month period spanning July 2014 to December 2015. Post-abortion family planning integration has doubled from 40% to 81%, and immediate postpartum family planning has grown from less than 1% at the initiation of the program to 21% during the past year.

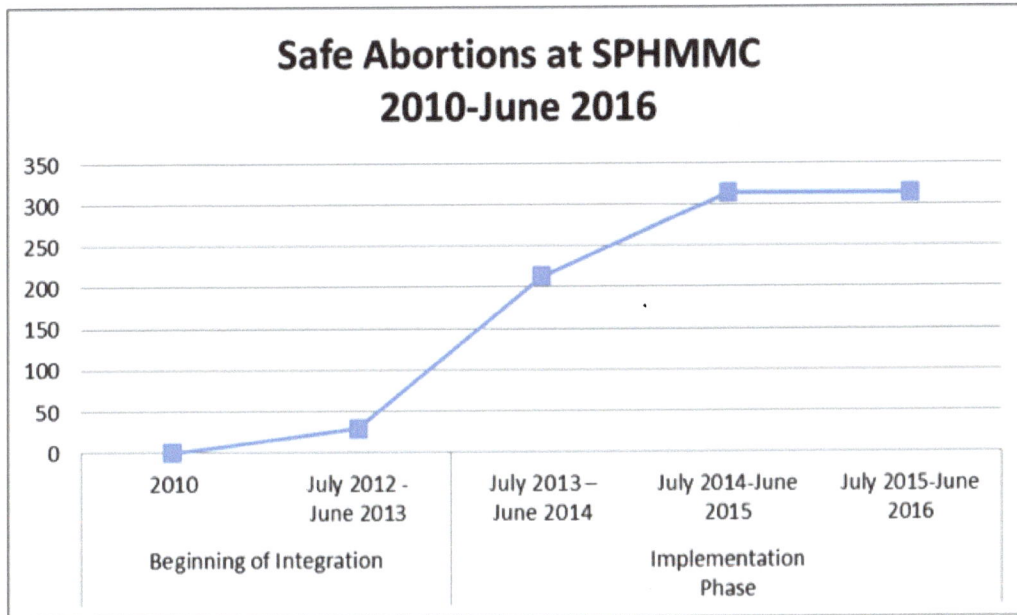

Safe Abortions at SPHMMC 2010-June 2016

Quality Improvement

When faculty from St. Paul's were doing observerships at the University of Michigan, they were learning not only new clinical knowledge and skills but also approaches of building a better health system, and they were inspired to bring a number of changes back to St. Paul's that did not require many resources. One of the biggest changes they made, which is now a hallmark of SPHMMC, is for OBGYN physician consultants to be on call, in-house, 24/7 as opposed to the previous policy of being *"on call"* to give advice mostly via telephone during off-hours and weekends and to only occasionally be called in when

ABORTION AND CONTRACEPTION SERVICES PROVIDED AT SPHMMC (2010–2016)

	Period	Number of Safe Abortions (SA)	Number of Safe Second Trimester Abortions	Post Abortion Contraception Provided (%)	Total LARC* Method Users
Baseline Period	2010	0	0	29%	Data Not Available
Beginning of Integration	July 2012–June 2013	29	0	40%	233
Implementation Phase	July 2013–June 2014	213	102	26%	1028
	July 2014–June 2015	314	262	81%	1736
	July 2015–June 2016	314	158	84%	2588

*LARC: Long Acting Reversible Contraceptives (Including Implants and IUDs)

complications arose. This has brought a significant improvement to both the quality of care and the quality of training delivered.

As part of its quality improvement (QI) initiatives, the OBGYN department has also put into practice a monthly family planning and abortion audit, which includes presentations and discussions that delve into the challenges of reproductive health service provision and accomplishments within the field, charting the way to better health service delivery.

TeamSTEPPS® training is an evidence-based set of tools aimed at optimizing patient outcomes by improving communication and teamwork skills among multidisciplinary teams of health care professionals. This training series was conducted by Dr. Sue Ann Bell, a faculty member from the nursing school at the U-M, for nurse and physician RH providers at SPHMMC, and it has improved the team approach in the care delivered. *"The integration is likely to empower midlevel staff as well when they see family planning being part of the training, as they can see its importance,"* says Dr. Feiruz Surur, chair of the OBGYN department at SPHMMC.

In addition, each OBGYN resident is expected to identify gaps in service delivery and plan and implement a QI miniproject to ameliorate the identified gap and improve quality of care. Accordingly, some of the QI miniprojects included preparing a family planning counseling checklist; guides to be used by antenatal care (ANC) and postnatal care (PNC) providers; preparing patient educational materials to be distributed by ANC and PNC providers, which included family planning information; and preparing a system to provide family planning commodities 24/7, just like emergency drugs. In addition to improving the quality of care, this process is expected to improve residents' problem identification and solving skills, enabling them to become stellar future leaders.

4. Supportive College Leadership

One of the pillars of the success of this program is the supportive SPHMMC leadership, beginning with Provost Dr. Mesfin Araya and Vice Provosts Dr. Lia and Dr. Tola, who created an environment that enabled the department to flourish and provided all the necessary administrative support to further boost the OBGYN department's growth in volume and quality and strengthened the partnership with U-M. This strong leadership in the beginning, and the visionary and bold leadership team that took over, led by Provost Dr. Zerihun, has directly impacted the success of the department by facilitating the recruitment of able OBGYN faculty from every corner of the country, reinforcing a culture of collegiality within the staff and faculty, and availing space and necessary equipment to expand reproductive health services within the premises of St. Paul's Hospital.

VI. Lessons Learned

Investing in the quality of training of future providers through this program of integrating family planning and safe abortion training into pre-service education at SPHMMC in partnership with the U-M has in a short period demonstrated that such an investment can bring multilayered changes. One of these early outcomes has been the development of competent and compassionate providers who not only can deliver comprehensive and much-needed services to women but also can take leadership to ensure those services are made accessible to women and are of quality. Implementing such programs in countries like Ethiopia, where around 300 OBGYNs are serving a country of 95 million, had its own challenges, one of which was the limited number of faculty in the department, especially at the initial phase of the program. However, most were overcome by a commitment for change, perseverance to overcome bottlenecks, and strong leadership at all levels.

Summary of lessons learned:

- The integration of contraception and safe abortion training to pre-service training in medical schools has done the following:
  - Demonstrated how this can be an opportunity to fully take advantage of trained physicians who give these much needed services in the primary health care system, as well as properly mentor and supervise lower and midlevel health providers in those facilities, improving access and quality
  - Enabled trainees who are enrolled in the school by giving them adequate time to gain deeper learning, understanding, and the right skills, including acquiring the right attitude to give care to women, hence creating a pool of health professionals who are also advocates committed to provide woman-centered care
  - Improved the quality of the training through its focus on simulation and skills-based training, creating strong competency and confidence in providing those services
  - Proved cost-effective compared to in-service training, where providers would have been taken away from their practice sites/facilities.
- Faculty development activities in clinical service, teaching, and research has, through the partnership with the U-M to implement this program, played a significant role in building a strong department that now has the capacity to fully run the program and be a leader in the quality of medical student and residency training and in the quality of clinical care they provide, as well as in their research outputs in reproductive health.
- Committed faculty and leadership at St. Paul's, coupled with the political commitment of the Ministry of Health, played a key role in ensuring the successful implementation of this program.

- The commitment of the faculty at the U-M to mutual and authentic partnership was instrumental to the development of the strong relationship between the two institutions that laid the foundation for an impactful and sustainable collaboration.

During a panel session at ICFP 2016, Dr. Ephrem Lemango, director of the maternal and child health directorate at the Federal Ministry of Health of Ethiopia said, *"Focus on pre-service academic programs highly complements the country's strategy of expanding the Health Extension Program, speeding up the achievement toward achieving the goal of reducing maternal mortality."* With the big strides SPHMMC is making in becoming a Center of Excellence in reproductive health nationally and regionally, it has demonstrated that a mutual and need-driven partnership between academic institutions, emphasizing building the capacity of the human resources and the infrastructure of the institution, is a model for sustainable development. Based on this evidence and the achievements thus garnered, this model is now being scaled up in eight other medical schools in Ethiopia through the Center for International Reproductive Health Training (CIRHT) at the U-M, with further plans to expand the program into other countries.

References

1. Ahmed, S., Li, Q., Liu, L., Tsui, A. O. Maternal deaths averted by contraceptive use: an analysis of 172 countries. *Lancet*. Jul 14 2012; 380 (9837): 111–125.

2. Canning, D., Schultz, T. P. The economic consequences of reproductive health and family planning. *Lancet*. Jul 14 2012; 380 (9837): 165–171.

3. Cates, W., Jr. Family planning: the essential link to achieving all eight millennium development goals. *Contraception*. Jun 2010; 81 (6): 460–461.

4. Cates, W., Jr., Abdool Karim, Q., El-Sadr, W., et al. Global development. Family planning and the millennium development goals. *Science*. Sep 24 2010; 329 (5999): 1603.

5. Cleland, J., Conde-Agudelo, A., Peterson, H., Ross, J., Tsui, A. Contraception and health. *Lancet*. Jul 14 2012; 380 (9837): 149–156.

6. Halperin, D. T. Scaling up of family planning in low-income countries: lessons from Ethiopia. *Lancet*. Apr 5 2014; 383 (9924): 1264–1267.

7. Olson, D. J., Piller, A. Ethiopia: an emerging family planning success story. *Studies in family planning*. Dec 2013; 44 (4): 445–459.

8. Abdella, A., Fetters, T., Benson, J., et al. Meeting the need for safe abortion care in Ethiopia: results of a national assessment in 2008. *Global public health*. 2013; 8 (4): 417–434.

9. Alkema, L., Kantorova, V., Menozzi, C., Biddlecom, A. National, regional, and global rates and trends in contraceptive prevalence and unmet need for family planning between 1990 and 2015: a systematic and comprehensive analysis. *Lancet*. May 11 2013; 381 (9878): 1642–1652.

10. Berhan, Y., Berhan, A. Causes of maternal mortality in Ethiopia: a significant decline in abortion related death. *Ethiopian journal of health sciences*. Sep 2014; 24 Suppl: 15–28.

11. Gebrehiwot, Y., Liabsuetrakul, T. Trends of abortion complications in a transition of abortion law revisions in Ethiopia. *Journal of public health*. Mar 2009; 31 (1): 81–87.

12. Guttmacher Institute. Facts on unintended pregnancy and abortion in Ethiopia. 2010; https://www.guttmacher.org/sites/default/files/factsheet/fb-up-ethiopia.pdf. Accessed May 10, 2016.

13. Prata, N., Gessessew, A., Campbell, M., Potts, M. *"A new hope for women"*: medical abortion in a low-resource setting in Ethiopia. *The journal of family planning and reproductive health care / Faculty of family planning and reproductive health care, Royal College of Obstetricians and Gynaecologists.* Oct 2011; 37 (4): 196–197.

14. Singh, S., Fetters, T., Gebreselassie, H., et al. The estimated incidence of induced abortion in Ethiopia, 2008. *International perspectives on sexual and reproductive health.* Mar 2010; 36 (1): 16–25.

15. Central Statistical Agency, Addis Ababa, Ethiopia, ICT International, Calverton, MD, USA. Ethiopia demographic and health survey 2011. 2012; http://www.unicef.org/ethiopia/ET_2011_EDHS.pdf.

16. Central Statistical Agency, Addis Ababa, Ethiopia. Ethiopia mini demographic and health survey 2014. 2014; http://www.unicef.org/ethiopia/Mini_DHS_2014__Final _Report.pdf.

17. Fortin, J. With Ethiopia: the U-M reaches around the world. *Medicine at Michigan* 2014; 16 (2).

18. Bekele, D., Nigatu, B., Fisseha, S., et al. Integrating family planning into pre-service medical training—early results from St. Paul's Hospital Millennium Medical College (SPHMMC). International Conference on Family Planning; 2013; Addis Ababa, Ethiopia.

19. Tadesse, L. Ensuring leadership in family planning and safe abortion: the role of medical education. XXI FIGO World Congress of Gynecology and Obstetrics; 2015; Vancouver, Canada.

20. Foreman, W. Ethiopia's foreign minister praises U-M's Ghana experience. 2014; https://michiganinethiopia.wordpress.com/. Accessed May 11, 2016.

21. Gebremeskel, B., Bekele, D., Tesfaye, A., Lemango, E., Hailemariam, M., Tadesse, L. Creating a continuum of care for Ethiopian women: integrating family planning and comprehensive abortion care into pre-service medical training. International Conference on Family Planning; 2016; Nusa Dua, Indonesia.

www.ingramcontent.com/pod-product-compliance
Lightning Source LLC
Chambersburg PA
CBHW052046190326
41520CB00003BA/211